Overeating

Understanding, Overcoming and Preventing Overeating, Binge Eating, Body Image Problems, Emotional Eating and Diet Troubles

Robert S. Lee

Table of Contents

Contents

The trademarks that are used are without any consent, and the publication of the trademark is without permission or backing by the trademark owner. All trademarks and brands within this book are for clarifying purposes only and are the owned by the owners themselves, not affiliated with this document.

Chapter 1. Eating Disorders and Body Image Issues in the United States

Everyone has a part of their body that they do not love and this is perfectly normal. The problem comes in when someone becomes obsessed with their physical appearance to the point that it is the primary focus of their life. It is very easy to become obsessed with your looks and your physical appearance because American culture is heavily focused on it. The media presents heavily touched up models and celebrities and delivers them as the ideal body type. Of course, these beauty standards are impossible to achieve, but the pressure to try and achieve it can trigger eating disorders and body image issues in both men and women of all ages.

When it comes to eating disorders and body image issues, there is not a single cause. However, research shows that the media and American culture's view on beauty standards does contribute. In some cases, this influence is not all bad. Here are some facts on how American media affects body image:

- Experimental and correlational studies show that the thin ideal that is constantly presented in the media is associated with internalizing the thin ideal, body dissatisfaction and disordered eating in women.
- Now, shows that primarily star African Americans seem to have a protective function. African American and Hispanic

women who watch these shows tend to have a higher level of body satisfaction.

- While adolescent boys do not seem to be very affected by media images, young men can develop a negative body image as a result.

- When it comes to women, young adults seem to be the most affected by the pressures of the media. They are most likely to develop body dissatisfaction and disordered eating as a result of media-imposed beauty standards.

- Men feel the most pressured to increase their muscle mass as a result of the focus on toned bodies in the media.

Research is still ongoing to determine the weight that the media carries in terms of eating disorders and body image issues. All that researchers know at this time is that it does play a role, but it is a small part of a larger issue. For example, issues like poor self-esteem, childhood trauma, family pressure and peer pressure also play into these issues.

Eating disorders and body image issues often go hand in hand, even when someone is recovering from an eating disorder. In the United States, it is estimated that as many as 24 million people, including both men and women, suffer from at least one eating disorder. Compared to all mental illnesses, the highest mortality rate is seen with eating disorders. It is also estimated that depression can be diagnosed in up to half of all people with an eating disorder.

There are several important things to know about body image that are helpful for those suffering and their loved one. Consider these

facts to learn more about negative body image
and how this affects people:

- Body image describes how a person
  thinks people see them and how they see
  themselves.
- Self-esteem and body image are closely
  related to one another. Low self-esteem
  can lead to body image issues and eating
  disorders, especially in teens and young
  adults.
- Eating disorders are common among
  those with body image issues and eating
  disorders can also contribute to a
  negative body image. This is a cycle that
  can be difficult to break.
- Up to 91 percent of women say that they
  have tried to diet at least once due to not
  being happy with their bodies. They
  often cite the media and peer pressure as

the primary reasons they felt the need to make changes to their bodies.

- Research shows that girls who find appearance most important also tend to watch a lot of television.

- Studies on women in college show that approximately 58 percent of them feel that they must achieve a certain weight.

- Approximately 20 percent of men and 40 percent of women say that they would consider plastic surgery to try and achieve their ideal body.

- Of all people who diet, approximately one-fourth will eventually develop an eating disorder in the future.

People ages 12 to 25 account for about 95 percent of people who have an eating disorder.

- When it comes to getting professional help for an eating disorder, only about

10 percent of people seek it out. Getting the right treatment in a timely manner is critical for proper treatment, the best chance at recovery and to minimize the risk of associated complications as much as possible.

As you can see, eating disorders and body image issues are not uncommon in the United States. Due to factors that drive them, everyone is at risk. It is important to understand these disorders because knowledge and the right support system are two of the most important preventative factors.

Chapter 2. Understanding Eating Disorders

Eating disorders are more common than most people think and they can be fatal. This is important to note because many people see them as a harmless habit. The following are the crude mortality rates for eating disorders, according to the *American Journal of Psychiatry:*

- 4 percent for anorexia nervosa
- 5.2 percent for eating disorders that are not specified
- 3.9 percent for bulimia nervosa

In general, eating disorders involve an extreme focus on food and negative feelings about body image. This causes people to develop habits that have significant health consequences. There are several types of eating disorders that you want to be aware of, with bulimia nervosa and anorexia nervosa being the most common. In fact, if you are just looking at people under age 18 in the United States, about one or two of every 100 will struggle with bulimia or anorexia. There are several factors that increase a person's risk of developing an eating disorder, including:

- **Being female:** Women of all ages are more prone to developing eating disorders compared to their male peers.
- **Family history:** Those with a close family member who had, or has, an eating disorder are at a higher risk.

- **Dieting:** People who tend to diet more frequently are more likely to develop an eating disorder.

- **Certain professions and hobbies:** There are certain professions and hobbies are more focused on weight and body types, such as sports and the arts. Being a part of these fields increases your risk of developing an eating disorder.

- **Age:** Those who are in their early 20s and teens are at the most risk.

- **Mental health disorders:** A large percentage of people who have eating disorders also have other mental health disorders.

- **Stress:** Significant stress can increase the risk of an eating disorder because it makes people feel like they finally have something that they can control.

Types of Eating Disorders and Their Symptoms

Most people are aware of anorexia and bulimia, but there are a number of eating disorders that you should know about. This is especially critical for those who are at risk for these disorders. The following are eating disorders to learn about:

- **Anorexia nervosa:** This disorder is characterized by severely restricting calories. Some people also exercise excessively and use various methods to purge. Significant weight loss, hair loss and a reduction in vital signs are common with this disorder.

- **Bulimia nervosa:** This disorder is characterized by eating large amounts of food and then purging it from the body via vomiting or using other methods, such as laxatives. Teeth rotting and stomach pain are common symptoms.

- **Binge eating disorder:** This disorder is characterized by often eating a significant amount of food, but not trying to prevent weight gain. Those with this disorder often gain weight quickly and may go on to develop conditions like high blood pressure and diabetes.

- **Eating disorder not specified:** This is an eating disorder that does not exactly fit the criteria of the disorders that are listed above. For example, atypical anorexia is in this category and it is a type of anorexia where the person's weight is not considered to be below what is normal. Another example is binge eating disorder where the person only binges occasionally. These are more difficult to diagnose because

the warning signs and symptoms are not
as apparent as they are with other types
of eating disorders. Other examples
include purging disorder and night
eating syndrome.

Causes of Eating Disorders

In most cases, several factors contribute to an
eating disorder. There is no single cause that is
directly associated with this disorder. The
following are the causes that have been linked
to all types of eating disorders:

- **Psychological and emotional
  health:** If someone has pre-existing
  issues in these areas, it can contribute to
  the development of an eating disorder.
- **Genetics:** Research shows that having a
  first-degree relative with an eating

disorder can contribute to developing this condition.

- **Society:** The pressure from peers and pop culture can contribute to someone developing an eating disorder.

Effects of Eating Disorders

All eating disorders come with a set of symptoms that generally indicate a negative impact on someone's health. However, there are also certain effects that can occur when someone has an eating disorder for a prolonged period of time. These effects can include:

- Significant health and medical problems
- Suicidal behavior or thoughts
- Relationship and social problems
- Anxiety and depression
- Development and growth problems
- School and work issues

- Substance abuse disorders
- Death

There are more specific effects that can occur with both bulimia and anorexia. These are typically related to not getting adequate nutrients due to having an eating disorder. With anorexia, be aware of the following:

- Drops in pulse, blood pressure and breathing rate
- No longer having a menstrual period
- Not being able to concentrate
- Feeling lightheaded
- Joint swelling
- Fingernails breaking and hair loss
- Soft hair growing on the body
- Anemia
- Brittle bones

With bulimia, be aware of the following:

- Constant stomach pain

- Tooth decay

- No longer having a menstrual period

- Kidney and stomach damage

- Chipmunk cheeks

- Losing too much potassium

Eating Disorder Warning Signs

There are signs that other people can see that may indicate that someone has an eating disorder or that they are close to developing one. You may not always be able to see these as a problem in yourself, but they tend to be very clear when you are looking at others. Look for the following warning signs if you suspect that someone may have an eating disorder:

- Only eating a few foods and removing entire foods groups from their diet

- Becoming emaciated and frail

- Constantly weighing themselves
- Excessive exercise
- Constantly feeling overweight
- Being lethargic, depressed and constantly cold
- Obsession with weight control and food
- Carefully portioning out food and counting calories before eating anything
- Withdrawing from anything that involves food
- Fearing weight gain
- Extreme unhappiness with body shape, weight and size
- Only eating foods that are low in fat
- Frequent use of diuretics, laxatives or enemas
- Immediately going to the bathroom after eating

Suspecting an Eating Disorder

When someone suspects an eating disorder, it is critical that it be diagnosed as soon as possible. The sooner a person starts to get treatment, the lower the risk of the more serious complications that can occur. An eating disorder diagnosis is made based on symptoms, signs and eating habits. Doctors will start by performing the following:

- **Psychological evaluation:** It is important to evaluate mental health since it is a major risk factor with eating disorders. Patients typically fill out a self-assessment and discuss their feelings, thoughts and eating habits with a mental health professional.
- **Physical exam:** To rule out other potential medical issues that could be

causing your symptoms, a physical exam is performed.

- **Other studies:** Your doctor will do things like lab work to determine the state of your overall health. This is critical since eating disorders often cause secondary health issues that need to be treated alone with the disorder itself.

There is a specific criterion used when diagnosing eating disorders that is set forth by insurance companies and mental health providers. Your doctor will review your symptoms and determine if they meet the diagnostic standards in the Diagnostic and Statistical Manual of Mental Disorders.

Treating Eating Disorders

Treating eating disorders require a multifaceted approach that involves a team of healthcare practitioners. You will generally work with your general practitioner, a dietician and a mental health professional. This ensures that all of the aspects of your eating disorder are treated properly.

Psychotherapy is very common because it helps you to take your unhealthy habits and replace them with healthy and productive ones. The following are common types of psychotherapy:

- **Cognitive behavioral therapy:** This is the most common type of therapy used for eating disorders, especially binge-eating disorder and bulimia. You will learn how to better track and recognize your moods and your eating habits, learn to cope with stress and develop effective problem-solving skills.
- **Family therapy:** For those who are younger, family therapy is often

beneficial for helping patients to recovery from an eating disorder. It works to involve the whole family in the recovery process so that the patient has the necessary support.

Nutrition education and weight normalization is an important part of treating an eating disorder. This is especially important for those who are either underweight or overweight as a result of their disorder. Your healthcare team will work with you to determine a healthy weight and create a nutrition plan to help you achieve this weight. This can be a lengthy process because it takes time to learn how to eat a balanced diet again. It is important to be patient and to keep up with the plan that has been created for you. Your plan will include a diet that has foods from all of the major food groups so that you get all of the nutrients that your body needs for optimal health.

Eating disorders cannot be cured by medications, but there are medications that can be helpful for some people when it comes to managing purging, binging or being severely preoccupied with food and eating. Since eating disorders may also be accompanied by other disorders like anxiety or depression, medications for these disorders may also be prescribed. Treating these disorders may help patients to make the changes necessary to recovery from their eating disorder and develop a better relationship with food.

In severe cases, some people have to be hospitalized to ensure proper care. This is typically done in cases of severe malnutrition. This allows doctors to restore nutrient levels and help you to get the calories that you need to recover. After hospitalization, some patients benefit from an outpatient program to help them stay on track with their recovery efforts.

Some people find it helpful to attend a support group with others who have eating disorders. This helps them to know that they are not alone. It is also helpful to discuss feelings and challenges with those who are able to understand them. Your doctor can often refer you to a support group in your area. How often the groups meet depends on the group, but they are generally once or twice a week. Ideally, people should go once a week to get the most benefit.

Part of treatment, is maintaining your treatment when you are at home. The following are helpful to enhance your doctor-prescribed treatment plan and improve your chances of recovery:

- **Keep up with your treatment plan:** Stick to your meal plans and make sure

that you attend all of your therapy
sessions.

- **Avoid isolating yourself:** It can be
easy to want to be alone while you are
recovering, but it is important that you
maintain a relationship with those who
are close to you.

- **Avoid weighing yourself:** When you
are recovering, the key is to improve
your relationship with food and improve
your overall health. Weighing yourself
can thwart your efforts and cause you to
fall back into old habits.

- **Talk to your doctor:** Your doctor will
be monitoring your health and making
sure that you are getting the nutrients
that you need.

- **Take note of your feelings:** Keep a
journal and write down what you feel.
This is especially important when it

comes to how you feel about your meals. You need to get these feelings out so that you do not harbor them. Holding them inside may harm your recovery by forcing you to maintain negative feelings toward food and eating.

Preventing Eating Disorders

There is no one way to prevent an eating disorder, however, there are a number of ways to reduce the risk. The majority of prevention involves what you can do for others, but these same methods can also be turned inward to help individuals to reduce their own risk of developing a disorder. The following are common preventative techniques:

- **Avoid dieting around children and encourage healthy eating:** This is important because when children grow up seeing constant dieting and a poor relationship with food, they are more likely to have similar issues as they grow older. Instead, make it a point to discuss nutrition, have your kids help you to prepare nutritious meals and snacks and eat together as a family as much as possible.

- **Create and help children maintain a healthy body image:** People come in all shapes and sizes and it is important to help children to embrace this. Never discuss your imperfections on front of your children. You want them to get a message of body acceptance from you, especially before they become teens. This will help them to build their self-esteem so that it is strong as they grow older and face peer and media pressures.

- **Talk to your kids:** Just like talking to your kids about things like drugs, you should also discuss body image and eating disorders. This helps them to understand how they develop and what the health consequences are.

- **Educate yourself:** Talk to your child's doctor to learn more about the warning signs so that you can identify any eating disorder or body image issues that your child may be experiencing.

Chapter 3. Eating Disorder and Body Image Issues Among the Different Genders

While eating disorders and body image issues are more common in women, men experience them too. Understanding how each gender is affected is important because this allows you to recognize problems earlier both in yourself and others.

Female Eating Disorder and Body Image Issues

Most women face a negative body image at some point in their lives. Women are prone to distorting their bodies, meaning that they see certain parts larger than they truly are. For example, a woman may feel that her thighs are too fat, but their thighs are perfectly in proportion with their body and everyone else sees this. Here are some facts about this:

- 40 percent of women see at least one area of their body as twice the size that it truly is
- 90 percent of women overestimate their body size by 25 percent

The majority of women feel that they need to be thinner at some point in their lives. This thought is what can trigger eating disorders, specifically when women become obsessed with the number of the scale. The most common eating disorders that women suffer from include anorexia, binge eating disorder and bulimia. Women are also at a higher risk for experiencing a related disorder called orthorexia. This condition is characterized by someone exercises obsessively to lose and control their weight.

Male Eating Disorder and Body Image Issues

Body image issues and eating disorders are far more common in women, but men experience these too. There are several differences in how these disorders affect men, compared to women. This can make body image issues and eating disorders more difficult to diagnose in men. In some cases, men are mistaken for simply taking an active role in their fitness instead of growing obsessed with their physique. This is especially true for men who are athletes because they naturally care about their health and their overall level of fitness. There are a number of facts that show how these issues affect men:

- Men generally do not feel pressure to be thinner. Men usually feel pressured to build muscle and become more fit. They want to develop six pack abs and increase the circumference of their biceps.
- Men may be muscular, but not see how muscular they really are, causing them to become obsessed with their muscularity. This can trigger an obsession with eating and using substances to try and increase their muscle mass faster than a proper diet and exercise will.

- Some men feel pressure to become more muscular based on the appearance of common childhood action figures. They see the build on these toys and want to look more like them because they see the toy's physique as ideal.
- The men who do feel pressure to become thinner are at a higher risk for depressive symptoms. They are also at a greater risk for binge drinking and drug use.
- Looking at high school boys in the United States who have body image issues, approximately four percent have taken steroids to try and improve their physique and build more muscle.
- Men who obsess over the size of their muscles are at risk for developing the disorder muscle dysmorphia. This is like body dysmorphia, but the sole focus is

on the amount of muscle mass. Men with this condition are at a higher risk of suicide and illegal substance abuse, including anabolic steroids.

- As many as four in every five men say that they have been unhappy with their body at least once in their life. 35 percent of these men say that in order to achieve their ideal body, they would give up a year of their lives.

- The following statistics represent the number of men suffering from an eating disorder: 0.3 percent have anorexia, 2 percent have binge eating disorder and 0.5 percent have bulimia.

Chapter 4. Body Dysmorphic Disorder

A focus on appearance is something that everyone has and looking your best is important. However, when someone starts to become obsessed with their appearance to the point where they are manufacturing flaws, the problem has already started. Body image is critical for good self-esteem, especially in young adults and teens. However, pressures from society can distort this image and cause conditions like body dysmorphic disorder.

Body dysmorphic disorder affects approximately one percent of people in the United States. While this is more common in women, both genders experience it. This disorder can become very serious so it is critical that treatment be started promptly. Knowing the facts about this disorder is critical for helping people to both recognize it and recover.

What is Body Dysmorphic Disorder?

Body dysmorphic disorder is considered to be a type of chronic mental illness. It is characterized by constantly thinking about your appearance and the flaws that you perceive are present. In most cases, the flaw is imagined or someone sees it as far worse than it truly is. For example, someone may have a scar that they are self-conscious about and see it as far larger and more pigmented than it truly is. This can reduce your confidence and cause you to obsess over it.

The flaws, whether real or perceived, take over your life and you spend hours each day obsessing over them. This can lead to other unhealthy behaviors, such as eating disorders, because of the need to try and fix the flaws, whether they can be fixed or not. This often takes over someone's life and makes it hard to do things like concentrate on work or school. As you continue to try and fix your flaw, you may make changes, but are never satisfied with them, resulting in further efforts to try and make changes that will not make enough of a difference to stop the obsession.

Typical Body Dysmorphic Disorder Behaviors

There are a few behaviors that people with this disorder commonly exhibit with the most common being compulsion and avoidance. Compulsion is a behavior that someone adopts when they are trying to alleviate tension that their obsessive thoughts are causing. For example, if someone has an obsession with their nose, they may constantly put on makeup or check their nose in the mirror. The behaviors of constant makeup application and mirror checking are the compulsions.

When someone has compulsions, they feel an irresistible or strong urge to constantly do them. When they give into their compulsions, they experience a sense of relief, but it is only temporary. This temporary relief allows the person to escape their bad thoughts or feelings. The compulsions tend to take up a lot of a person's time because they typically have to be repeated multiple times throughout the day in order to help the person find some comfort.

Avoidance behaviors are also common and they can lead to serious issues like isolation. For example, someone may perceive a flaw as so bad that they stop leaving the house because they feel so ashamed of it. They may stop going to classes, stop looking in mirrors and stop socializing just to try and avoid their flaw.

The compulsive actions, avoidance and obsessive thoughts become a pattern with this disorder. The relief that these behaviors provide is only temporary. In fact, the more a person practices avoidance behaviors or performs compulsions, the more often they need to do these to get relief. It becomes like a drug and to continue to feel the high, they have to do these behaviors more and more. The longer a person has these behaviors, the harder it is to break them and return to healthy behaviors.

What Causes Body Dysmorphic Disorder?

Experts do not know exactly what causes this disorder. They believe that there are a number of factors involved that change a person's perception of their appearance. Some theories include:

- **Genes:** There is research that shows that when someone has a family member with this disorder, they have a higher chance of developing it at some point in life.

- **Brain differences:** Experts believe that those with this disorder may have differences in their brain chemistry and brain structure. The brain chemical most associated with this disorder is serotonin. Serotonin imbalances are linked to other mental illnesses too.

- **Environment:** Someone's life experience, environment and culture may play a role in them developing this condition. This is especially true if someone has experienced negative things about their self-image or body image.

In addition to the believed causes, there are also certain risk factors that appear to make it more likely that someone will develop this disorder, including:

- Having a family member with this disorder
- Having low self-esteem and certain other personality traits
- Having depression, anxiety or another psychiatric disorder
- Childhood teasing and other negative life experience

- Societal expectations of beauty or pressure

How this Condition Affects a Person's Life

Body dysmorphic disorder can have a significant impact on a person's life. It can cause issues like social isolation and anxiety. Understanding the impact that this disorder can have is critical for being able to recognize it if it occurs in you or in someone that you know.

There are a number of symptoms associated with body dysmorphic disorder that can significantly impact a person's life. Severity varies based on the person, but the symptoms have the potential to become worse with time for all people. The symptoms of this disorder can include:

- Being preoccupied with physical appearance
- Believing that you have an appearance defect that everyone views as ugly
- Extreme self-consciousness
- Constantly looking in the mirror or completely avoiding them
- Avoiding social situations
- Needing constant reassurance about your appearance
- Believing that everyone sees you as unattractive
- Having multiple cosmetic procedures done, but never being satisfied with the results
- Feeling the need to wear a lot of makeup or grow facial hair to cover up flaws
- Staying home to avoid being seen in public
- Excessive grooming

- Not wanting to be in pictures
- Constantly comparing your looks to those of others

There are certain features that people tend to obsess about when they have this disorder. While someone can obsess over any feature, the features most commonly targeted include:

- Facial features, including complexion, acne, the nose, lips and wrinkles
- Vein and skin appearance
- Genitalia
- Hair, such as baldness and thinning
- Muscle tone and size
- Breast size

In many cases, the feature that someone is obsessing over is not a negative flaw. This disorder simply forces them to see the feature in a negative light. People can reassure the person that there is nothing wrong with the feature, but they never believe it. The obsession over the feature can control someone's life to the point where it causes them to stop going to school, work or out with friends and family. The person puts so much effort into focusing on this flaw that they are unable to be productive doing anything else.

If this disorder goes untreated, there is the risk for several complications that can significantly impact a person's life. The potential complications of this disorder include:

- Social isolation and social phobia
- Trouble going to school or work
- Repeated hospitalizations
- Suicidal behaviors or thoughts
- Obsessive-compulsive disorder
- Lack or close relationships
- Low self-esteem

- Mood disorders or depression
- Anxiety disorders
- Substance abuse
- Eating disorders

Another potential complication is having unnecessary cosmetic surgery to try and fix the flaw that someone is obsessed with. Every surgery comes with a set of risks that can further cause problems, and in some cases, cause permanent health issues. Those who start having cosmetic procedures are at risk for finding new perceived flaws to obsess over, resulting in this condition getting worse and more widespread.

Getting Help for Body Dysmorphic Disorder

The first step in getting help is to get an accurate diagnosis so that you can receive the proper treatment for this disorder. This is not an easy condition to diagnose, so it is common for doctors to do a number of tests before making a diagnosis. The following are commonly performed to rule out other conditions, check your overall health and work toward making an accurate diagnosis:

- **Physical exam:** Your doctor will want to assess your overall health and determine if there is a physical condition causing your symptoms.
- **Psychological evaluation:** This involves assessing your psychological health to determine if you are experiencing a mental health disorder, such as body dysmorphic disorder.
- **Lab testing:** This will help to rule out other possible conditions and determine

if this condition has affected your physical health.

The next step is pinpointing the exact disorder that you are experiencing. This involves exploring the diagnostic criterion used to diagnose this disorder. Your doctor will use the Diagnostic and Statistical Manual of Mental Disorders to determine if your symptoms align with the symptoms of this disorder. The criterion that doctors are looking at include:

- Severe preoccupation with a minor flaw or imagined defect in your appearance
- Your appearance obsession taking up so much of your time that it inhibits your ability to be productive and function normally

Getting medical treatment is critical for the best chance at recovery. Treating this disorder is not easy and it is important that the patient is willing to go through the treatment and recovery process. There are two primary treatments that doctors use to help patients recover, including cognitive behavioral therapy and medications. In most cases, people are prescribed a combination of the two to alleviate the disruptive behaviors and help you to change your behaviors and your mindset so that you are able to recovery.

Cognitive behavioral therapy works in a number of ways. Those going through this therapy will work with a trained therapist to focus on:

- Building the tools that you need to stop the negative thoughts that appear to automatically occur. This allows you to view yourself in a way that is more positive and realistic.

- Learning how to better socialize with others and adopting other healthy behaviors.

- Learning more about body dysmorphic disorder, as well as your thoughts, behaviors, feelings and moods.

- Developing healthier ways to manage your rituals or urges.

Medications are commonly used for this condition, but there is not a specific medication that treats or cures body dysmorphic disorder. Doctors usually choose medications that treat conditions like anxiety or depression because they may help to balance serotonin levels. Serotonin is a brain chemical that is thought to play a role in this disorder. The medications can help to reduce the behaviors that are common with this condition so that you are able to make the right changes and resist issues like avoidance behavior, preoccupation with your appearance and compulsions.

Selective serotonin reuptake inhibitors, also known as SSRI medications, are the most commonly prescribed. They work to balance serotonin levels to alleviate your symptoms and improve your overall mood. They may also help to control repetitive behaviors and obsessions in those who have this disorder. Compared to other antidepressant medications, this class of drugs tends to be the most effective, according to current research. You will usually start with a low dose and gradually have it increased until the medication is producing the desired results. Like all medications, there is the potential for side effects so it is important that you keep all of your appointments so that adjustments can be made if necessary.

There are certain other medications that doctors may prescribe to those with this condition. For example, some people with this disorder also experience delusions. In this instance, an antipsychotic drug may be prescribed to control the delusions. Those taking an antipsychotic drug also usually take an antidepressant as well since both drugs are used to control different aspects of this disorder. Make sure that you maintain all appointments and let your doctor know if any medications are causing side effects that are too unpleasant to manage to allow for adjustments to improve your quality of life.

In the most severe cases, people may need to be hospitalized to ensure proper treatment and safety. In this case, the person spends time in a psychiatric hospital so that their healthcare team can closely monitor them and develop a treatment plan that will be effective. This is generally recommended when the person is a danger to themselves or when they are unable to properly care for themselves. How long someone needs to stay in the hospital is highly individualized, with some people needing to stay for a few days and others needing to stay for weeks or months. After a hospital stay, it is common to receive outpatient treatment that continues to build on the treatment that you received in the hospital.

There are many things that doctors often recommend that their patients do at home to enhance their treatment. These promote recovery and work well as a complement to your traditional therapies. The following can be added to your doctor-prescribed treatment:

- **Maintain your treatment:** It is important that you never miss an appointment with your doctor or a therapy session.

- **Learn more about body dysmorphic disorder:** When you understand the facts about this disorder, it makes it easier to understand the purpose of the treatments that are prescribed to you. This increases the chance of compliance with the regimen.

- **Get active:** Many people with this disorder can benefit from regular exercise and physical activity. This can help to reduce the effects and prevent the weight gain that can worsen this condition. Check with your doctor before increasing your physical activity to ensure safety. If you are new to exercise, consider something relatively easy, such as walking or swimming.

- **See your doctor regularly:** You should see your doctor approximately once per year to check up on your overall health. If you are feeling under the weather, see your doctor to determine why.

- **Take all medications exactly as prescribed:** It is important to take your medications exactly as your doctor prescribes them. In many cases, doctors prescribe medications like antidepressants to help manage this disorder. Abruptly stopping these medications can worsen your condition or cause unpleasant withdrawal symptoms. If you are taking a medication that is causing uncomfortable side effects, talk to your doctor. They can usually adjust the dose or help you switch to another medication to reduce side effects while keeping you current on your medication regimen.

- **Know the warning signs:** As you go through treatment, you will learn about the factors that can trigger your behaviors. Knowing your warning signs helps you to take control over them so that their effects are not so severe. When you are able to take control, your triggers will not be able to cause you to back track in your recovery.

- **Avoid alcohol and drugs:** Those with this condition are at a higher risk for drug and alcohol abuse. Due to this risk, it is important to avoid them during and after your recovery.

During your recovery and throughout your life, there are certain things that you can incorporate into your daily life to help you stay on track and not experience a relapse. These activities will help you to maintain a positive body image, as well as improve your overall health and outlook on life. These activities include:

- **Start writing in a journal:** It is important to be able to express your emotions and get them out so that they are not able to get bottled up. A journal is a safe place where you can be completely honest about your feelings and emotions.

- **Take care of yourself:** It is important that you consider your overall health and take the time each day to ensure that you are as healthy as possible. You want to do things like exercise regularly, eat a healthy diet and get plenty of sleep each night.

- **Join a support group:** You may find it helpful to discuss your condition with those who understand what you are going through. Your doctor can help you to find a body dysmorphic disorder support group in your area.

- **Make decisions when you feel good:** If you are feeling distress or despair, avoid making important decisions. This is because you want to make sure that you are making decisions when your head is clear so that you can properly think them through.

- **Do not allow yourself to become isolated:** It can be hard to stay social when you have this disorder, but it is critical. Spend time with those you love and take advantage of positive social situations.

- **Check out self-help books:** Your doctor or therapist may have some self-help books that they can recommend to help you learn coping strategies.

- **Know your goals and stay focused on them:** When you are recovering from this disorder, you will find that it is an ongoing process. When you keep your goals in mind, it makes it easier to stay motivated.

- **Practice stress management and relaxation:** It is important that you are able to properly control your stress levels since stress can trigger this disorder. Things like tai chi and yoga are things that you can do daily to keep yourself calm, relaxed and centered.

There is no way to completely prevent this disorder from happening. However, it is known that most people develop this disorder during their adolescent years. Because of this, it is critical to promote a positive body image and self-esteem in young children. This gives people the tools that they need to avoid the triggers that can cause body dysmorphic disorder. This same strategy can also help to prevent a relapse in those who are recovering from this condition.

Chapter 5. Developing a Positive Body Image

When you have a positive body image, this reduces the risk of developing an eating disorder or problems with your body image in the future. The key is understanding why your body is what it is and how to learn to embrace your individual beauty. Remember that everyone is beautiful and everyone has many positive traits that help them to contribute great things to the world. No one loves everything about their body, but when you work on accentuating your favorite parts, you will quickly stop concentrating on the parts that you do not like. This allows you to be happier and more comfortable in your skin.

Understanding How Genetics Influences the Body

The size and shape of your body is highly dependent on your genetics. Genetics even influences your body weight. This is why no two bodies are alike. You inherit a set of genes from each of your parents and these come together to create the personal traits that you have throughout your life. It is important to know this because it is important to know that there is only so much that you can do to change your body. You want to focus on your overall health and how you feel physical and emotionally. When you are healthy, you are typically able to do the following:

- Keep up with your daily responsibilities because you have enough energy to do so

- Spend time with your friends and family
  without feeling physically or emotionally
  strained
- Concentrate on work and school without
  difficulties or constant lapses in your
  ability to focus
- Participate in physical activity and
  sports without getting overly exhausted
  or easily winded
- Sleep well at night and feel good when
  you get the right amount of sleep
- Able to eat enough calories each day
  without difficulty or feeling guilty about
  it

Talk to your doctor and make sure that you see
him or her on a regular basis to keep an eye on
your health. Most people only need to get a
physical exam once a year to stay up-to-date on
their health. Your doctor will help you to

determine if you are at a healthy weight for your age, body type, general health and height. This is what is important since being overweight or underweight can lead to significant consequences. If you need to gain or lose weight to reach the right weight for you, talk to your doctor to ensure that you do it in a healthy and balanced way.

Lastly, avoid comparing your body to celebrities, your family and your friends. Your body is unique to you. The following are ways to ensure that you are as healthy as possible with your body type:

- Eat a well-balanced diet that properly incorporates all of the major food groups
- Be respectful to your body
- Get moderate exercise on a regular basis, balancing strength, cardiovascular and flexibility training for optimal fitness

- Get enough sleep every night so that your body is well-rested

- Take the time to relax and express your feelings for optimal mental health

Steps to Developing a Positive Body Image

Having a positive body image is something that you strive for and work for. There are many things that you can start doing right away to improve your body image and your overall outlook on your life. Start doing the following every day to feel better about yourself and your body:

- **Appreciate your body's abilities**: Your body can do extraordinary things and appreciating these can help you to better love the body that you live in. Think about things like running, jumping and even breathing. These are very complex and your body allows you to do them with little to no effort.

- **True beauty goes below the surface:** Your true beauty includes all aspects of you, not just your physical appearance. Beauty is really just how you feel and you should never allow anyone to influence how beautiful you feel. Practice self-acceptance, be confident and be open. This all comes together to help you see that your beauty starts on the inside and radiates outward.

- **Keep positive people at your side:** When you are constantly around people who are positive, you will naturally become more positive too. This allows you to better focus on the positive things in your life so that the negative things do not take over and influence how you feel about yourself.

- **Dress for your body:** There is not a single person on the planet that looks great in all of the latest fashions. Find out your body type and work with it. There are plenty of great things that will look amazing on your body. The next time you head out to do some shopping, try on clothes in the store and take a trusted friend with you. Make sure that this friend will give you honest and kind feedback so that you can choose the best clothes for your body.

- **Do something nice for you:** At least once a week, do something nice for yourself. This could be grabbing a sweet treat, taking a bath or taking a walk by yourself. As long as this is something that you enjoy, it will help you to relax and feel your best. It will also make you happier so that there is a lesser chance of developing a negative body image.

- **Make a list of your best traits:** Everyone has a number of positive traits and reminding yourself about what these are helps you to improve your body image. Make a list of 10 things that are awesome about yourself. You can carry this around with you and when you start to feel down on yourself, grab the list and look it over. This gives you an instant boost of confidence and helps you to better focus your thoughts on feelings on what is truly important.

- **Check out the whole person:** You are not just your weight, hair color or how you dress. You are a whole person and it is important that you look at yourself as a whole. This allows you to become more aware of all of the positive traits that you have.

- **Shut out the negative voices:** Everyone has a voice inside that is far too critical and you want to shut this voice out. Take your negative thoughts and turn them around by drowning them out with positive thoughts.

- **Avoid what makes you feel bad:** You surely have a few triggers that make you feel bad or put you in a negative mood. Identify what these are and work to avoid them. It is usually not possible to avoid them completely, but you can reduce your exposure to them. For example, if a certain website makes you feel negatively about your body, avoid visiting it and make sure that it is not in your browser's bookmarks.

- **Help others more:** When you take the negative energy that makes you feel bad about your body and spin it into something positive, this naturally boosts your confidence and your body image. Take a few hours a week to volunteer, take opportunities to help your friends and family or do something to clean up your community and make it a better and cleaner place for yourself and your neighbors.

Chapter 6. Preventing Body Image Issues

When it comes to body image issues, prevention is critical because everyone is at risk. Even if you do not have a history of negative body image or eating disorders, there is still a chance that your perception of your body image could change in the future. There are a number of preventative strategies that you can start using today to prevent this. There are also several techniques that you can use to help others to maintain a positive body image. Remember that a good support system is the number one way to keep yourself and others positive and healthy.

Be a Role Model for Others

Being body positive is one of the best ways to promote a positive body image in others. This also helps you to better appreciate all of the positive assets that you personally possess. Consider all of the following to promote a positive body image by being a role model for yourself and others:

- **Examine your own thoughts and beliefs:** To be an effective role model, you have to have strong convictions. This means that you have to look at your beliefs, specifically how they relate to your body and your relationship with food, and make solid decisions so that you can help others to do the same thing.
- **Have a positive self-image:** It is important that you make it clear that you accept your body as it is. Be gracious

with compliments and focus on the attributes that you feel most confident about.

- **Improve your relationship with food:** Make sure that your diet is non-restrictive and well-balanced. This allows you to help others to do the same thing. It also ensures that you are healthy and getting all of the nutrients that your body requires.

- **Express your feelings:** Never hold things in because this can contribute to body image issues and problems with food. If you are experiencing difficult emotions, learn how to express them in a productive manner.

Learn More about Body Image

Being knowledgeable about body image is important because you need to be able to recognize problems as they occur. This is beneficial for both you and those who can benefit from your help. You want to know how body image issues manifest in both males and females and what some of the warning signs are. This gives you the opportunity to take charge and help to prevent the more severe issues before they have a chance to begin.

Know about issues like peer pressure and media pressure and how these contribute to body image issues and eating disorders. You also want to explore the issues that most affect those in your age group and the age group that you spend the most time with.

There are a number of other factors that can contribute to body image and eating disorders, including:

- Pre-existing emotional and psychological health issues
- Low self-esteem
- Feeling like you have no control in life
- Trouble expressing your feelings and emotions
- Troubled personal relationships
- Feelings of inadequacy
- Unrealistic views about what is beautiful
- Experiencing discrimination associated with your ethnicity or race

Be Sensitive to Outside Causes

Body image issues and eating disorders typically stem from multiple causes, including those that do not seem to be related. For example, changing schools is something that everyone does at some point, such as going from middle school to high school. For most teenagers, this is a normal part of life and the impact is minimal. However, for others, this is a major transition that impacts them significantly. They may feel pressure to make major changes to try and fit in this new environment, triggering issues with food and body image.

There are times when someone's coping mechanism is their body image issues. This is typically triggered by additional underlying issues, but the fact that they are using this as a coping mechanism has to be addressed first. This gives you the chance to peel back the layers and identify the underlying causes.

Preventing Body Image Issues in Athletes

Athletes, especially teen athletes, are a group that is particularly prone to body image issues and disordered eating due to the pressures associated with making weight and overall performance. There are several things to consider when you are an athlete or working with athletes to help improve their body image and work to prevent future issues, including:

- Promote the love of the sport over winning or weight control. This is especially important in sports that put a lot of emphasis on weight like wrestling, swimming and gymnastics. Show things like sportsmanship and concentrate on overall performance. These play a bigger role when it comes to success and this must be emphasized.
- Be clear that there is more than just the sport. As a team, spend time together outside of the sport, such as with team dinners and outings. This alleviates the in-team competition to help improve the

relationships of the athletes. This gives the athletes something more positive to concentrate on.

- Never put emphasis on things like weight restrictions. Certain sports do have weight classes, but never try to pigeon hole an athlete into one weight class. Make sure that they have the training to compete in all weight classes so that they have options and do not feel the need to focus on their weight.

- Understand the right nutrition for athletes. Athletes need more calories and more of certain nutrients. Having this information helps athletes to develop a positive relationship with food and it helps them to put emphasis on healthy eating.

- If you feel that you are having issues with body image or disordered eating, talk to your coach. If you are a coach, make sure that you are available to your athletes and that you understand how to help them if issues like this occur so that you are able to provide the right help before things get very serious.

Chapter 7. Overcoming a Negative Body Image

Once body image issues set in, it can seem like they will forever have a hold on you, but this is not true. You can make the right changes to overcome a negative body image, but be patient because the changes do not happen overnight. The key is to start working on the changes today and you will start to see changes in how you view yourself and how you feel about your body. There are a number of ways to overcome a negative body image and you should start with one because you do not want to try and make several changes at once because this can leave you feeling overwhelmed.

Be kind to yourself and others. This is the first thing you may want to start with because overall kindness will change your perspective on life and your body. When you see another person, look deeper than their outward appearance. When you start to see others for who they are, you will notice that you start to focus more on who you are inside too. This takes the attention off of any of the physical characteristics you have that you are not happy about.

Put it all into perspective. As a person, you are far more than just your body. Your body is simply what houses you. Focus on your family, your accomplishments, your hobbies and the other positive aspects of your life. Everyone does many things very well and you will see this when you sit back and reflect on it. To put it simply, ditch the mirrors and the scales and take out a pen and paper. Write down all of the positive things in your life and then put them list somewhere where you will see it often throughout the day. You can also place one by your nightstand so you see it when you wake up every morning.

Forget about dieting. Dieting often causes fear and negative emotions so eliminate this word from your vocabulary. You simply want to live a healthy lifestyle. When you put a healthy lifestyle in a diet bubble, there is a failure rate of about 95 percent and when you fail, this further feeds into your body image issues and increases the risk of eating disorders.

Accept your body. As you learned in a previous chapter, genetics have a major impact on the shape and size of your body and there is very little you can do to change your genetic traits. For example, if your father has broad shoulders or your mom has wide hips, you may too and there is no way to change this. It is important that you work toward accepting these traits and focusing on the areas of your life that you do have some control over.

Listen to your body. This takes practice because it is not always easy to know what your body is trying to tell you. Keep note of what is happening when your body feels a certain way. For example, if you feel tired, think about how you have been sleeping or when you are having trouble focusing, think about things like your stress level and sleep quality.

Set healthy and realistic goals. It is easy to set goals that are very ambitious because in today's society everyone wants to get things quickly. However, since ambitious goals are very hard to achieve, this can create problems in the future. When you create realistic goals and meet them, this furthers your ability to overcome the negative body image issues that you are dealing with. As you meet your health goals, you will gain confidence and start feeling better about yourself. You can work with a nutritionist to get started so that you can get advice along the way.

Do not look at celebrities for body inspiration. When you see a celebrity in a magazine, remember that they are digitally enhanced and that they are not perfect. They too have flaws that they are working to embrace. When you are working on your body image, it is important that you focus solely on yourself and your individual needs. Comparing yourself to celebrities, or anyone else for that matter, will make you feel worse since no two people will look alike. In fact, even identical twins usually have at least one very small difference, such as one have slighter thinner hair than the other.

Celebrate your beauty. Even when you have a negative body image, you surely have a few traits that you do love about yourself. Maybe you love your eyes, hair or smile. Consider the traits that you love and accentuate these. This will improve your body image because it changes your focus to the traits that make you feel confident. Women can play with makeup or different hairstyles. Men can try new hairstyles or facial hair patterns. These are fun and new and will help you to make small changes that make you feel great about yourself.

Get the help you need when you need it. When you are feeling bad, reach out to someone you trust and talk about it. If you are trying to improve your health, get a buddy that can help you to create and achieve your realistic health goals. You have people in your life that want to help you because you are important to them. Never be shy about approaching them, whether you just want to talk or you need more complex help. Keep in mind that you can also get help from people like your doctor, a personal trainer, a nutritionist or even a teacher that you trust. The key is to know when you need help and to reach out and get it so that you never feel alone.

As you can see, body image issues and eating disorders are not uncommon, but there are many things that you can do to reduce your risk and help those who you care about. Maintaining good health, surrounding yourself with positive people, learning about these disorders and working to improve your confidence are good ways to prevent these issues. If you ever feel that you are developing a disorder or you suspect that a loved one is in trouble, it is important to get the right help right away. Early treatment can work to prevent the more serious complications and reduce the amount of time it takes to recover and restore your health.